NAYLA BYXBE

THE CARNIVORE DIET: A PERSONAL EXPERIENCE

Quest for Optimal Health

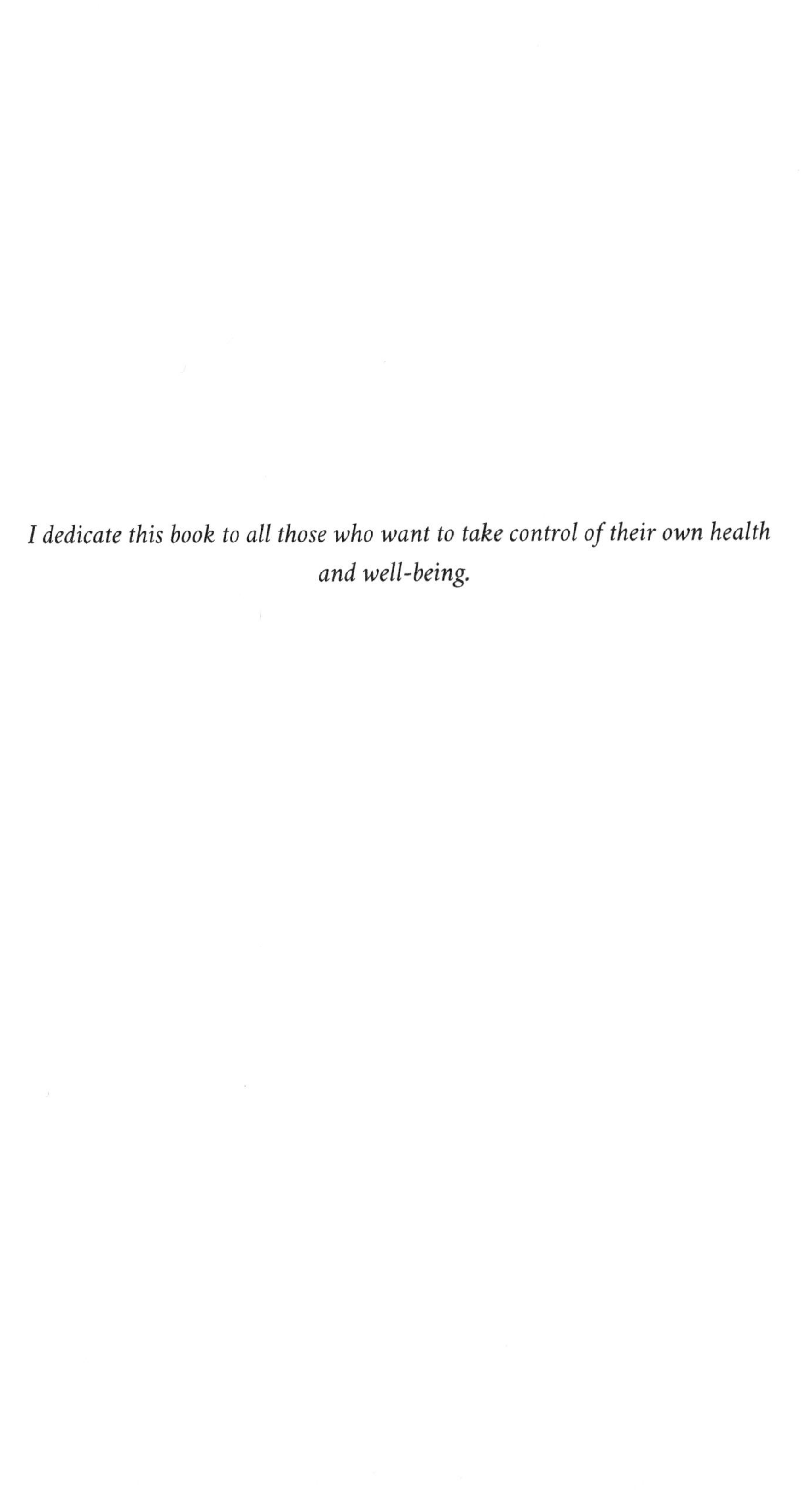

I dedicate this book to all those who want to take control of their own health and well-being.

"The doctor of the future will give no medicine, but will interest his patients in the care of the human frame, in diet and in the cause and prevention of disease."

Thomas Edison

Contents

Acknowledgement   iii

  1 INTRODUCTION   1

  2 WHAT IS AYURVEDA?   3

  3 ANTI-AGING AND LONGEVITY SUPPORT   4

  4 WHAT I WAS HOPING FOR   5

  5 KETO AND ME   6

  6 THE CARNIVORE DIET   7

  7 WHEN YOUR KIDS BECOME YOUR TEACHER   8

  8 HOW I STARTED   9

  9 MY YOUTUBE GURU RESOURCES   12

 10 MY RESULTS: 90 - DAY CARNIVORE DIET CHALLENGE   14

 11 WHAT IS B B B E?   15

 12 CARNIVORE AS THE ULTIMATE ELIMINA-
     TION DIET   17

 13 MY FOOD CHOICES   18

 14 WHAT I EAT IN A DAY   20

 15 CHALLENGES I ENCOUNTERED ALONG
     THE WAY   22

 16 THINGS I DIDN'T EXPECT   24

 17 A FEW SPECIALTY ITEMS I RECOMMEND   26

 18 INTERMITTENT FASTING IS FUN   27

 19 BUTTER: I Want to Talk about Butter   29

 20 A FEW RECIPES   30

 21 KEEP IT SIMPLE   33

22 SUPPLEMENTS THAT I USE   35

23 WHAT ABOUT EXERCISE?   37

24 OVERVIEW OF CARNIVORE DIET   38

25 CONCLUSION: GETTING HEALTHY IS FUN   40

26 WHAT'S NEXT FOR ME IN CARNIVORE DIET?   41

27 WHAT'S NEXT FOR YOU?   42

Epilogue   43

Acknowledgement

I want to thank my friends and colleagues who encouraged me to share this.

1

INTRODUCTION

I am very excited to share this information with you. I have recently succeeded in completing a special carnivore 90 Day diet Challenge. All along the way people have been interested and asked me to share in detail how I was doing it. They wanted it for themselves and felt like they needed more details and didn't know where to find it. I have been very happy to share with one person at a time; however, this was becoming a regular occurrence. I was inspired to create a small book and include space where they could add and keep their own notes as they journeyed through their own experience.

I have spent the most of my professional life in the field of health, wellness and well- being. My journey in this field began in the operating room on the "cutting edge" as a Surgical Technologist. I learned so much from the wonderful surgeons with whom I had the privileged to work with. They were generous with their knowledge and loved to teach those who were interested. I could not have learned what they shared with me from a textbook. What they brought alive for me was the thought process that drives me to this day. That thought started with thinking, "There has to be a better way"! Western medicine is wonderful!

Of course, I'm grateful for it and use it as needed, but it is not my first "go to". I have been passionately interested in my health: how to get healthy, how to stay healthy and how to teach others to do the same.

My journey took me deep into Ayurveda healthcare. I graduated from the California College of Ayurveda in Grass Valley, CA in 2005. During my one year internship after graduation I was hired as a teaching assistant for their long distance Ayurveda learning program. I went on to develop a successful practice in my hometown, Redding, CA. I accepted a position to continue to practice Ayurveda at the International Sivananda Yoga Retreat in Nassau, Bahamas. My passion was en kindled to address the root cause of disease, that being cellular inflammation due to an unhealthy diet and lifestyle. I continued to be open to receiving new information, and the Carnivore Diet and lifestyle came into my awareness.

2

WHAT IS AYURVEDA?

I want my reader to know what Ayurveda means. Maybe you have never heard of it before now. For those who have not, Ayurveda means Knowledge and Life. It is the Art and Science of Life and Longevity. This is a science that is over 2000 years old and viable to this very day. Ayurveda addresses the root cause of disease, which is cellular inflammation.

I'm seeing that today's technology is opening up the mysteries of these ancient truths, allowing us to take control of our own health. Ayurveda teaches that food is medicine.

It also teaches that plants will poison humans when they are used inappropriately or, I could say, disrespectfully. This comes from a story straight out of the Vedas, the ancient Ayurveda writings. When I first heard it, I didn't understand it. When I heard one of my favorite carnivore diet experts teaching how plants can poison us, I got it! It goes completely against the way we have been taught in the Western world and it is hard for us to take in. Just keep an open mind and lean into this Carnivore Diet idea with me.

3

ANTI-AGING AND LONGEVITY SUPPORT

Eating meat is anti-inflammatory for the systems of the human body and eating a high carbohydrate diet increases inflammation.

Reducing cellular inflammation allows for gene expression to self regulate. This study is at the forefront of the quest of today's medical scientists! That's pretty exciting to me.

Our body can heal our DNA which will then allow our gene expression to self-regulate and the effect is optimal health, anti-aging and increased longevity. This has my attention and maybe yours too.

4

WHAT I WAS HOPING FOR

I wanted to feel better! I wanted to get my strength, stamina and vitality back. I wanted to feel alive and productive again. I wanted to lose weight and get my body back and love it again. My mind was sluggish, and I was feeling confused. I had anxiety, high blood pressure and some chronic kidney disease going on. Oh, and high cholesterol! My doctor had sent me to a cardiologist. His great news was to offer a second blood pressure pill and a Statin. I had my own idea and ran it by him. I was going home to try the Keto Diet for 90 days. He agreed to my plan and would hold off on the medication.

5

KETO AND ME

To be fair, I didn't put much effort into the idea or study of Keto. I had a loose idea. Measuring and balancing the protein-to-fat ratios and carbohydrate counting was not on my bandwidth. Consequently, I gained weight! Why was I surprised? The Keto Bars were just another cookie in my cupboard, and the Keto Ice Cream was sublime! Cravings were a severe problem for me. Hindsight, it was those carbs! When I was feeling like "Eeyore " Keto was not a safe place for me! Carbohydrates cause inflammation and insulin spikes. I needed something different.

6

THE CARNIVORE DIET

J ust to be clear, the Carnivore Diet is an animal based diet. We only eat meat from any ruminant animal. Ruminant refers to an animal that chews a cud; cows, goats, lamb, bison, elk, deer, etc. Bacon and fatty parts of pork, (fatty chicken and fatty fish (especially salmon) and sardines are included as protein sources. **NO seed oils, vegetable oil, canola oil or Crisco.** We can have bacon grease, tallow (i.e. rendered fat) and butter. Lots of butter, eggs, water and salt.

We do not take in **any** carbohydrates. This is a **zero carb** diet. So when you might be choosing a meat that is processed like sausage, check the label. Look for no sugar added and carbs less than 1,that is what we looking for.

We eat to **satiation** at every meal. No snacking, make sure as Dr. Barry says, "Eat till you are comfortably stuffed".

That is the diet. No measuring food, counting calories, micros or macros. Eat when you are hungry to comfortably stuffed and stop. Eat again only when you are hungry. No snacking.

7

WHEN YOUR KIDS BECOME YOUR TEACHER

I discovered The Carnivore Diet when my son was preparing for a bodybuilding competition. He was sharing with me this crazy diet his trainer put him on. One morning he called me and said he just had 12 eggs for breakfast and how he was 'leaning out', which is his way of saying his muscles were showing. His body was in ketosis, and his fat was being used as fuel. When the body builder removes fat, the muscle stands out. I started researching this diet and found a growing crowd in the carnivore community. All kinds of people were participating in this diet and experiencing tremendous results. For me, it felt right and I was willing to give it a try. I give a lot of credit and gratitude to my son because he opened this door for me and totally supported me!

8

HOW I STARTED

1. I educated myself by researching mainly on YouTube. I found leaders in the carnivore community that were making huge impacts in the medical world.

2. I started gradually by making small changes. I focused on reducing carbohydrates thinking it would help me to ease into this change.

3. MINDSET!!!! You've got to have the right mind set....COMMITMENT! Without *commitment* all you have is a wish!

4. I set my goal and committed to 30 days of the Carnivore Diet. I intended to start at the beginning of the month.

5. I decided I would do 30 Days and evaluate where to go from there. I kept hearing Dr. Ken Berry saying that anyone can do something for 30 days. His words planted the seed that I would go all the way.

6. I got two large calendars and a planner. I wanted my accountability calendars to be in places where I would see them all the time.

7. I gave myself a star at the end of every day as a reward for completing the day with no cheating! Stars and Happy stickers motivated me. Imagine your calendar all filled up with rewards for succeeding, every single day.

8. I weighed every morning and documented on my calendars and planner.

9. I got a special notebook. I encourage you to do the same. Make it fun!

10. I took some before pictures.

11. I saved my old jeans that got too baggy as a reminder.

12. I wore my skinny jeans until they became baggy, and I'm saving them as a reminder.

13. I was open to one day at a time.

14. This is key to my success. I found my favorite supporting YouTube educators and subscribed to their channels. This kept my YouTube feed full of positive supporting videos.

15. I watched **YouTube Carnivore** videos **everyday.** I made this my daily study and I shared what I learned.

16. I created a folder in my YouTube library of my favorite videos making it easier to find and share with others.

17. I asked questions on YouTube in the comment section if I had any

challenges I wasn't sure how to handle. My experience was that people were welcoming and willing to share.

18. I learned when I 'subscribed and liked' the videos that it supported the creator of the content and helped the community to grow.

19. I shared with my doctor that I was going to do the Carnivore Diet for 30 days. She totally supported my decision.

20. I asked her for some blood tests so we could keep track of the changes. I highly suggest you do that for yourself. It's a great "point A to point B" as you track your success.

21. I didn't cheat.

22. I didn't quit.

9

MY YOUTUBE GURU RESOURCES

Dr. **Ken D Berry** is a leader in this community. He has a great library of videos and interviews to choose from that is available to watch and share.

Dr. Sarah Pugh is a Quantum Biologist and Justifies carnivore diet using SCIENCE. She is interviewed by Joey Schwartz @Thebusysuperhuman.

 Anthony Chaffee MD is a great educator and offers many interviews with other doctors.

Dr. Bright is an impressive DO physician. I believe she is a Canadian.

Dr. Shawn Baker is a podcaster you won't want to miss.

Dr. Lisa Wiedeman has a great video regarding sweeteners on Keto. She is an OD.

Myzerocarblife, Kelly Hogan has not eaten plants in 12 years and has been on the Carnivore Diet 12 years. She is a motivator and leader in the community, a great resource. She lost 120 pounds eating the Carnivore Diet and healed herself of boils, acne and obesity.

Steak and Butter Gal coaches and focuses on BUTTER. She eats sticks of butter.

5 Minute Body is another leader in the community.

Check out the video **The Carnivore Diet:Why Does It Work So Well? "Plants are trying to kill you!"** This video is 12.42 minutes long.

Ketogenic Woman, shares recipes on her cooking show. She is excellent at both Carnivore, BBBE and Keto. She is a valued resource.

Carnivore Quest is a couple, Larry and Cassie, on their Carnivore quest to lose two hundred pounds, between them. They share from their hearts and have created a very supportive community.

Two Crazy Ketos are a man and wife doing a podcast. It is fun, relatable, educational and motivational.

Laura Spath shares her weight loss on the Carnivore Diet.

10

MY RESULTS: 90 - DAY CARNIVORE DIET CHALLENGE

Completing a 90 Day Carnivore Diet Challenge was amazing for me. No cheating and never wanting to quit was a new experience. After eating my first meal I was so happy. My hunger was satisfied and cravings were a thing of the past.

What I loved most was the release of weight. I lost 24 pounds and my clothes size was reduced by 2-3 sizes.

I have more energy! My attitude is resilient again. My blood pressure is normal. My doctor is not worried about my cholesterol and my kidneys even smiled with a lower number.

I love myself. I said yes to self-love and self-respect. I can say no to others if it is not good for me. I empowered myself to level up.

11

WHAT IS B B B E?

WHAT IS BBBE?

When we say, "BBBE" it means: Beef, Bacon, Butter, Eggs. Inside this acronym, Beef stands for all the ruminant animals. The BBBE Diet is a more specialized version of the Carnivore Diet and consists only of Beef, Bacon, Butter, Eggs salt and water.

The Challenge of 30-90 days is a program where the newbie or chronically ill person is encouraged to check this out for themselves. Giving a time frame gives you a starting date, a middle and an ending date. The mind is much more willing to play along.

Regarding *Redmond's Real Salt: this salt is mined in Utah from an ancient dry sea bed. This sea salt is not contaminated like our oceans, nor does it have micro plastics, common to other choices of salt. This salt actually has the unique quality to have a post digestive effect of cooling. Regular table salt has a drying and heating post digestive effect. This is a healthier choice.

Dr. Ken D. Berry created this diet and has several videos on this subject if you need more clarity.

12

CARNIVORE AS THE ULTIMATE ELIMINATION DIET

If you have autoimmune disorders or chronic inflammatory conditions you might have been advised to consider an elimination diet. In my experience, it is difficult. This ancestral diet will bless your body with relief and restoration in a pretty simple way.

By choosing to eat only Carnivore, you are eliminating ALL carbs. Red meat is an anti-inflammatory food. Carbohydrates are inflammatory. Removing carbohydrates reduces inflammation and allergic reactions that you are aware of and those that you are not yet aware of.

Now you may be mourning the loss of all those wonderful things nature provides and you are rethinking this whole idea. Don't be afraid. When your health improves and the fat disappears along with your symptoms, you will be able to add back into your diet one food at a time. Start with the one you miss the most. Your awareness and sensitivity will be so acute you will know if it is safe for you or not.

13

MY FOOD CHOICES

You may not be familiar with all of these. I wasn't either and only learned as I got hints from the community and then visited my local butcher market. The local butcher is very happy to share his knowledge on his products.

1. Bone In Rib eye
2. Baked Bone Marrow....elegant treat!
3. New York Steak
4. Hanging Tenders....very rich red cut
5. 80-20 grass-fed hamburger
6. Beef Short Ribs
7. Wagyu Short Ribs, extra marbled/fatty
8. Chuck Roast
9. Pork Belly, better than bacon
10. Bacon...lots of it
11. Sausage , sometimes, not often
12. *Redmond's Real salt! very important
13. Eggs, organic and free range

14. Butter, my favorite is Irish Gold, salted
15. Coffee (not after April 1) herbal tea, maybe
16. Water, Pellegrino
17. Salmon
18. Cream cheese
19. Chicken, dark meat with skin on

14

WHAT I EAT IN A DAY

I'm at day 90, and, frankly, I don't eat that much to report about, and I'm good with that. But you need to know what it might look like starting out. Typically, I eat between 11 AM and 1:30 PM, that's when I break my fast. Bacon is on my to do list. I love it and eat as much as I want. It is always a treat. The fat content is very satisfying. I learned to poach eggs by cracking them straight into the boiling water and cooking for 3-4 minutes. Put them into a bowl with butter and enjoy. Burger patty with eggs is another option for breakfast time. I prefer to eat my second meal within a six hour period of my first meal. No snacking. My favorite meal is Bone-in Rib eye, rare. Tip: eat several bites of the delicious fat first. By taking the fat in first it primes your system to fat burning mode. Note, I have never chosen to eat fat before, but when I experienced the satiation that fat gives and my cravings mysteriously disappeared, I dropped that old notion. You will understand completely.

I drink plenty of water! Electrolytes are a staple on this diet and plenty of salt on my food. Dr. Ken Barry will remove any fears you may have around the evils of salt.

I drink S.Pellegrino mineral water and find it very satisfying.

21

15

CHALLENGES I ENCOUNTERED ALONG THE WAY

1. Felt the urge to snack: Here's what I did. I made sure I was hydrated. I ate some butter. I I reflected on if I took in enough fat with my meal. My 'go to' is eating some cool salted butter.

2. Craving: I encountered this after a business trip where I had some terrible burger patties, several days in a row. What I needed was quality meat and for me that is rib eye steak. I feel the reason the burger patties didn't work for me was that they didn't have enough fat in it. That is why the rib eye was calling me. I started experiencing cravings when I was into the third month. I checked in with the Community and the consensus was to increase my fat intake.

3. Leg cramps! Oh,yeah! Magnesium, potassium and sodium (also known as ELECTROLYTES) are essential on this diet, and I found my favorites. LMNTS.COM (more on this later).

4. Coffee - Yes? No? Only 1 cup of coffee a day! Suggestion: It's good with Butter whipped into it in the morning. Dr. Ken Berry says drinking more than one cup of coffee will interfere with your body's true hunger signal. He also said drinking excess water will do the same thing.

5. A 5 day seminar in another state with flights, long connections and driving to location. I ordered carnivore. They did the best they could. I brought along sardines just in case I had no choices. Fortunately, I left them all there. Those are not my food of choice. but, I'm committed and would have done it. I hear a 3 day fast on sardines is a needle mover for weight loss. Just passing information. Food for in flight times I found packaged olives to be so satisfying along with bacon chips I prepared in the air fryer!

6. Eating in Restaurants. It gets easier. Order from the side menu. Order the burger patty and carefully explain to your waiter that you only eat meat and that means no veggies, no bread, no garnish and no seed oil! You will taste the seed oil if they use it. I strongly suggest you politely send it back if that happens. Here is the reason why. Seed oil has a ½ life of 4 YEARS. That means it takes your body 4 years to get that out of your system. This is an opportunity to self honor your body and your word/commitment.

7. Constipation: I was concerned about that since I believed fiber was necessary. I stayed the course and my body did adjust and now I experience natural healthy elimination. Dr. Ken Berry has videos on all these issues. Go check it out. Be fearless.

16

THINGS I DIDN'T EXPECT

- I didn't expect to see the belly fat disappear.

- I didn't expect to see my fat go and my body to remodel and restore so well.

- I didn't expect to have the clarity of mind and increase in self-control.

- I didn't expect to feel satisfied with a diet and never cheat in 90 Days.

- I didn't expect to be thrilled with my body appearance ever again.

25

- I didn't expect the Carnivore Diet to assist my life's trajectory as much as it has.

- I didn't expect to discover the ancestral diet to be as far reaching as it is.

- I didn't know I would feel so strong and full of energy.

- I just didn't know, and now I do.

17

A FEW SPECIALTY ITEMS I RECOMMEND

An Air Fryer is a must. I chose the Ninja brand. It's a great price and doesn't take up too much room. Plus, it travels well.

A large cast iron skillet for braising, Cassey's braised chicken soup and braised chuck roast. This is still on my bucket list.

Milk frother to whip up the butter coffee.

32 oz water bottle for the electrolyte drink.

Immersion Blender

Scratch protected thongs for the air fryer.

18

INTERMITTENT FASTING IS FUN

Fasting and Intermittent Fasting is a large subject and many books are written about this topic. They cite all the health benefits and all the different ways of fasting. Our body goes into fasting naturally when we are sleeping. Our body goes into a fasting mode with our last meal of a day. We 'break' that fasting period when we take in our first food of the day.

Hopefully, we do not eat in the middle of the night, as that interrupts our bodies natural resting and cleaning time. Eating late in the evening and in the middle of the night is unhealthy and it causes weight gain.

Consider how long you sleep and when you break your fast with eating. That might be 8-10 hours where your body was not working to digest food. When we stretch this time of not eating and digesting food, our body gets to repair and stay in ketosis burning our stored fat.

The simplest way to ease into longer periods of time is to simply wait an extra hour before you have your "breakfast" in the morning. When you are ready, another option is to stop eating earlier in the evening by an hour. Then you will have accomplished intermittent fasting for 10 to 12 hours! You will quickly notice the results of increased energy; clarity and enthusiasm will spark your carnivore journey. I have found holding off taking in food till around 11 AM or 1:30 PM gives me more time and more energy in the working hours of the day.

There is a lot of conversation around **what breaks** the fast. Eating will wake up your digestion. The taste of sweetness will trigger insulin and end your fast. Even chewing gum will break your fast. Dr. Ken Berry gives a great talk on this subject. He does say 1 "coffee experience" is okay and will not break your fast. He says adding butter is okay and frothing it will make it taste better.

I used intermittent fasting whenever it appears the scale is stuck. My maximum fast was 48 hours and when I returned to eating the pounds I lost never came back. Recently I ate steak and noticed the next morning it felt heavy in my stomach. I decided I needed to fast and let my body rest. It felt obvious that I had plenty of nutrition on board and eating was not necessary.

19

BUTTER: I Want to Talk about Butter

BUTTER: I Want to Talk about Butter

I had to open my mind around "eating butter". In this community the butter conversation is loud. We are not talking about eating margarine. That would be gross. That is what I related to it too. So, slowly, I took a nibble and slowly I received the blessing. It satisfied my body; my cells were jumping up and down like it was getting Spring Rain after decades of drought. Butter and fat have been demonized, and this diet will prove it to you. Enjoy the many benefits of eating butter as our ancestors did. Internal cell hydration that will reflect on your face and skin.

20

A FEW RECIPES

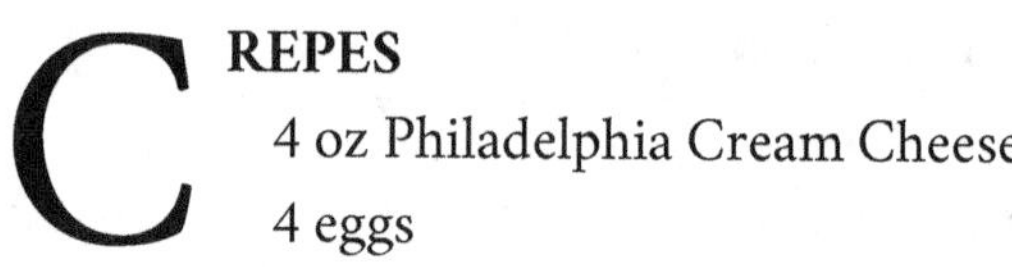

CREPES
4 oz Philadelphia Cream Cheese
4 eggs

Use an immersion blender to beat together until all the cheese is mixed in, no chucks, and frothy.

Into a medium-high heat non-stick pan, pour about 4 tablespoons of batter into the buttered non-stick pan. Let it cook about 3-4 mins until it browns and flip, cook for about another 3-4 minutes. Fill with a little bacon and scrambled egg or sausage and egg....so yummy.

HAMBURGER SOUP

Boil marrow bones to make a broth. This takes time. A slow cooker might be suitable.

Cook up your hamburger (80-20) till done. Spoon into a soup bowl the amount of hamburger you want and cover with the bone broth. Satiating! You will feel the goodness.

AIR FRY Rib eye Steak

You can take a frozen steak and put in an air fryer on "roast" and cook for about 11 minutes on each side. The roast feature on the frozen meat will create a crust and keep the meat juicier. Salt after cooking. Salting before cooking toughens the meat.

SNACK TIME: PORK BELLY

Air Fryer…preheat 4 minutes on air fry

Cut up pork belly into little bits. Put in a preheated air fryer and cook till golden brown.

Put in a bowl or small plate and salt. Munch time and delicious fat.

BUTCHER FRIEND: ASK YOUR BUTCHER FOR STEAK TRIMMINGS!

These are trimmings from Rib eye and NY Steaks.

Cut them up like the pork belly and cook on ROAST setting in the Air Fryer till done.

I buy a couple pounds at a time as some cuts don't have enough fat.

Fat trimmings also can be rendered for your cooking. Pour it off into a clean jar that you can put a lid on to store in the fridge

AIR FRIED BEEF SHORT RIBS

Wash short ribs and dry with a paper towel. Salt with Redmond's salt. Let meat come to room temp if possible.

ROAST setting in the air fryer creates a crust, keeping the meat juicy.

BACON

Cooking bacon on Roast will keep it from drying out. Dr. Ken Berry has a great video on bacon.

BACON WRAPPED MEATBALLS

80/20 Hamburger: MAKE form into small meatballs, wrap with bacon. Secure with toothpicks and roast in an air fryer or oven.

Options:

1. Poke a hole into a meatball, place a dab of cream cheese and close then wrap bacon and cook.
2. Cover soft boiled egg with hamburger, wrap with bacon, secure with toothpick and roast.

These are great for packing lunches.

21

KEEP IT SIMPLE

I believe it was Dr. Ken Berry who created the idea of BBBE. He wanted to make it simple and memorable. Beef, Butter, Bacon, Eggs, water and salt.

He said when you think you're hungry and have the options of beef, bacon, butter, and eggs to choose from, you will go one of two ways. If you are hungry, these options are inviting. You would say, yes, to these nutritious dense foods. If you aren't really hungry, and just looking for some satisfaction, you will turn away from them and desire sweet or salty snack treats and you would eat mindlessly and not be satiated.

When you are eating the carnivore diet you will be able to sense which department is trying to get your attention and it will be easy to make the better choice and nourish your body.

You may have noticed my recipes and food list looks pretty simple. I do like to cook and I do like simple things. If you LOVE to cook let me reassure you that you can get as fancy as you want. The Ketogenic woman is all about cooking and creativity. Go join her YouTube and have a ball. We get to choose how we want to do this diet and lifestyle. Above all else, make it fun.you want. The Ketogenic woman is all about cooking and creativity. Go join her YouTube and have a ball. We get to choose how we want to do this diet and lifestyle. Above all else, make it fun.

22

SUPPLEMENTS THAT I USE

A question that is often raised by the people new to BBBE is (can I take supplements?") The Answer is yes. Here is my list that I love having in my wellness plan.

LifeVantage TriSynergizer : Nrf2, Nrf1, NAD

LifeVantage, Rise AM with micronutrients

LifeVantage, Reset PM with micronutrients

LifeVantage, D+3 with micronutrients

Trace Minerals, *Beef Organs 500mg
   *My choice is to take a supplement of beef organs because I do not want to eat these organs. Maybe someday, but not right now. Thank goodness for having a choice.

ELECTROLYTES

Taking electrolytes is talked about a lot. I didn't take action on it until the muscle cramps started happening. I'm giving you the heads up, this is a must do. I chose the product LMNT! Visit drinklmnt.com/quiz and find what meets your individual needs. Plus they offer you a free full size packet with a purchase. Money back offer if you are not satisfied and you keep it..no mailing it back. Daily use, pre-workout and study too!

23

WHAT ABOUT EXERCISE?

When you first begin it is advised you do not exercise. I did because I had already started working with a personal trainer and didn't want to stop.

I finally stopped and discovered that I could have lost more weight from the beginning had I not been exercising.

Now I do it again because my weight loss is almost at my goal and I want to build my muscle mass. My body has been properly nourished and it feels like a natural and smart move for me. That's what my body told me. I trust my intuition. Besure to take your electrolytes when exercising.

24

OVERVIEW OF CARNIVORE DIET

Our ancestors ate a meat-based diet. Meat was sought out first because it was nutrient-dense and had life preserving value. They "feasted on the kill" to satiation. Eating was about surviving and with abundance they could thrive. Meat and fat were the focus. They ate from nose to tail, organs, muscle, bones, marrow and fat. They wasted nothing. What they added to their diet was dependent upon location, season, and availability.

We have evolved and have availability of foods from all over the world despite our location, climate or season. We have switched our dominant food to be plant-based, refined, manufactured, processed packaged foods. We replaced the animal fats with seed oils and turned the food pyramid upside down with meat and fat being reduced to the lowest value. Then disease began to rise to the epidemic levels that we see now. Humans are sicker than ever before, and we can change this.

This Ancestral Diet, Carnivore, is also referred to as "The Proper Humane Diet". For those keeping an open mind and wanting to take control of their own health it is recommended to do this diet for 30

Days and test results for yourself. Going for 90 Days, 3 months, will give you even better results. If you have chronic diseases or health issues, lean into the 90 Days. This will give your body time to reset, and you can consciously move forward.

25

CONCLUSION: GETTING HEALTHY IS FUN

The Carnivore Diet is so different, and that made it fun for me. Not knowing what I could really expect brought about a daily interest in this project.

At this point I want to share some motivational thoughts that I feel inspired to say.

Be curious. The Carnivore Diet is simple and requires less time in meal prep. A satiated body will naturally eat less and less often. You can say good-bye to old paradigms that keep you sick, fat and stuck. Say yes to something new. Start your health journey and create a long health span. Be brave. Go all in. That doesn't mean "cold turkey". Plan, prepare, educate, commit. Stay connected to community and positive support and go!

I'm excited for you and those you love as you get healthy beyond your wildest expectations! I did and you can too!

26

WHAT'S NEXT FOR ME IN CARNIVORE DIET?

You may wonder if I am choosing to quit after the 90 days. I have decided to continue going forward. I know for myself this is a lifestyle that works for me and serves my highest good, optimal health! My next step commitments are:

#1. Caffeine Free starting APRIL 1, 2023.

#2. Carnivore Diet **EXTENDING** to 180 days. I will use this simply as a marker. I heard that the Carnivore Diet will self-regulate your ideal weight. I am about to see for myself.

#3. I am committed to including salmon on a weekly basis. I think I can do it with bacon.

27

WHAT'S NEXT FOR YOU?

I would love to hear all about it.

Thank you so much for joining me.

It is my hope that you will try the Carnivore Diet for yourself and share it with your family and all those that you love.

If this little book has helped you I would deeply appreciate it if you would leave a favorable review on Amazon.

Epilogue